SCHIZOPHRENIA AND MULTICULTURALISM

POEMS FOR CHARITY

I0104972

By Moeze M Lalji

'One million people commit suicide every year'
The World Health Organization

Moeze M Lalji

Published by
Chipmunkapublishing
PO Box 6872
Brentwood
Essex CM13 1ZT
United Kingdom

http://www.chipmunkapublishing.com

Edited by Steven Hoy

About the Author

My name is Moeze Lalji. I was born in Uganda in 1958 and came to England as a refugee in 1972. I was a paperboy in my school days, then I went to Leeds Polytechnic, then I worked for a small firm of chartered accountants, then I worked for a bank, then I and my wife owned a sub-post office business and worked for a property company; after that I had my breakdown and I now suffer from schizophrenia. I also come from a back ground of mental health.

I have one daughter and with my wife they are my strength. I belong to the Ismaili community and my faith is in the Aga Khan that is keeping me alive and the obvious support from the mental health team.

Moeze M Lalji

SCHIZOPHRENIA AND MULTICULTURALISM

HER MAJESTY THE QUEEN

(I SENT THIS POEM AND THE QUEEN
APPRECIATED MY POEM BY LETTER
RECEIVED FROM LADY IN WAITING)

Dear Lord

I have found you

Dear Lord

Hazar Imam

Opened the door

And let me in

Dear Lord

Hazar Imam

Reminded me

My day on earth

Confused with Her Majesty The Queen

Dear Lord

Hazar Imam

Said read

Moeze M Lalji

BUCKINGHAM PALACE

28th March 2007

Dear Moeze,

The Queen wishes me to write and thank you for the poem which you have sent for Her Majesty to see.

The Queen thought it was kind of you to send her this and much appreciated your message of good wishes.

Yours sincerely,

Susan Hussey.

Lady-in-Waiting

Moeze Lalji

SCHIZOPHRENIA AND MULTICULTURALISM

HER MAJESTY THE QUEEN

H=House of Mother she represents

E=Excellent are her ways

R=Respect her for holding the forte

MAJESTY

M=Many years a mother stays

A=All say many things to her

J=Just watch her heart

E=Excellent is her heart to listen

S=Soon she will advise you

T=Take her not for granted

Y=You can make the mistake easily

THE

T=Tradition she represents

H=Hold on to your mother

E=Excellent she is

QUEEN

Q=Question her

U=Understand to Question her

E=Excellent mother will go

E=Excellent forte will go

N=Never will you replace an excellent mother

Dear Lord

You said learn from

Hazar Imam

The Heaven shall open

Amen

IN MEMORY TO H M QUEEN ELIZABETH THE QUEEN MOTHER 🌹

Dear Lord 🌹

I have found you

Dear Lord 🌹

Hazar Imam

Opened the door

And let me in

Dear Lord 🌹

Hazar Imam

Reminded me

My day on earth

Confused with H M Queen Elizabeth The Queen Mother

Dear Lord 🌹

Hazar Imam

Said read

H M QUEEN ELIZABETH THE QUEEN MOTHER 🌹

H=Her real name is mother of all mothers

M=Mother she is excellent

QUEEN 🖋

Q=Question not her experience

U=Understand the experience passed down

E=Excellent is this experience

E=Excellent is this experience

N=Never can it be replaced

SCHIZOPHRENIA AND MULTICULTURALISM

ELIZABETH

E=Every tradition offers

L=Light of evolution

I=Important symbol is light of evolution

Z=Zindaghi is evolution

A=Always the grace comes out

B=Bowing down the children to this grace

E=Every child learns grace

T=There you see blessings

H=Held in Queen mother's hands

THE

T=Touch her for blessings on the country

H=Hold her for blessings on the country

E=Excellent are these blessings on the country

QUEEN

Q=Quietly our Queen mother looks everywhere

U=Understand what she sees

E=Excellent is what she sees

E=Excellent is what she sees

N=Now gently see her to see what she sees

MOTHER

M=Mother is always earth

O=Only she understands what she holds

T=Taking every community in her hands

H=Holding them like babies

E=Every cry and footstep she hears

R=Respect is all we have for our Queen Mother

Dear Lord

You said learn from

Hazar Imam

The Heaven shall open

Amen

MULTICULTURALISM -PLURALISM

Dear Lord

I have found you

Dear Lord

Hazar Imam

Opened the door

And let me in

SCHIZOPHRENIA AND MULTICULTURALISM

Dear Lord

Hazar Imam

Reminded me

My day on earth

Confused with Multiculturalism - Pluralism

Dear Lord

Hazar Imam

Said read

Multiculturalism – PLURALISM

M=Many Are Our Ways

U=Understanding Has Accepted This

L=Life Comes From Many Backgrounds

T=Tensions Arise When It Is Rejected

I=Important It Is To Value It

C=Contribution Should Be Taken

U=Under Each Culture

L=Life Becomes Meaningful

T=To Address Their Needs

U=Under Democracy

R=Respect Should Be For Each Culture

A=All Needs Under Democracy Cannot Be Met

L=Life Gives Limited Budget

I=Important Priorities Have To Be Met

S=So Being Patient Is Important

M=Many Things Have Been Achieved

PLURALISM

P=People Are Diverse

SCHIZOPHRENIA AND MULTICULTURALISM

L=Like A Garden Of Flowers

U=Understanding Circumstances

R=Respecting Circumstances

A=All Contribute To Unity

L=Life Tries To Cater For Each Rose

I=Important It Is For Democracy

S=So The Budget Is Limited

M=Many Things Have Been Achieved

Dear Lord

You said learn from

Hazar Imam

The Heaven shall open

Amen

BRITISH VALUES TAKE FOR GRANTED

Dear Lord

I have found you

Dear Lord

Hazar Imam

Opened the door

And let me in

Dear Lord

Hazar Imam

Reminded me

My day on earth

Confused with British Values Take For Granted

Dear Lord

Hazar Imam

Said read

BRITISH VALUES TAKE FOR GRANTED

B=Best They Are At Systems

R=Respect They Have For Systems

I=Important Is Systems

T=They Identify All Needs

I=Important Is Life

S=Search Life To Understand

H=Have It Documented Open To All

VALUES
V=Very Much Respect For Tradition

A=Always Have Your Say

L=Let Your Frustrations Out

U=Understand Democracy

E=Every Culture Is Respected

SCHIZOPHRENIA AND MULTICULTURALISM

S=So Much To Learn From Them

TAKE

T=Their Good Deeds Are Many

A=Always Looking After Their Citizens

K=Keep Them Educated

E=Every Opportunity They Have To Learn

FOR

F=For You Have Worked Hard

O=Only Looking For Solutions

R=Respect You Have For Human Rights

GRANTED

G=Go And See Other Countries Children

R=Respect You Will Have For Your Country

A=And You Will Appreciate

N=Nearly All The Blessings

T=That You Take For Granted

E=Every Crime You Will Stop

D=Democracy Should Be Shown By Visiting The Unfortunate

SCHIZOPHRENIA AND MULTICULTURALISM

Dear Lord

You said learn from

Hazar Imam

The Heaven shall open

Amen

A TALK WITH MY PSYCHIATRIST

Dear Lord
I have found you
Dear Lord
Hazar Imam
Opened the door
And let me in
Dear Lord
Hazar Imam
Reminded me
My day on earth
Confused with A Talk With My Psychiatrist
Dear Lord
Hazar Imam
Said read
A Talk With My Psychiatrist
A=All Of Us Have Different Personalities
TALK
T=Take My Wife's Personality

SCHIZOPHRENIA AND MULTICULTURALISM

A=Always Good At Communication

L=Lively When She Talks

K=Keeps The Truth Lit

WITH

W=When She Speaks

I=It Is Out Of The Heart Straight

T=Truth Is All She Likes

H=Has No Feelings How You Will Feel

MY

M=My Personality Is Sensitive

Y=You Find Me Best In Writing Words

PSYCHIATRIST

P=People's Feelings I Think Of First

S=Slow Are Things With Me

Y=Yet For My Wife Things Move Fast

C=Catches Feelings Fast

H=Has The Sign Of Libra

I=Important Is Justice To Her

A=Allah Demands A Balanced Scale

T=Take My Star Sagittarius

R=Respect I Have For Many Thoughts

I=Important It Becomes To Know Everything

S=Sensitive Means I Also Get Hurt Very Quickly

T=Talim I Am Learning To Be Assertive But Slowly Says Psychiatrist

Dear Lord

You said learn from

Hazar Imam

The Heaven shall open

Amen

ANGELS GIVE A TOUR OF HEAVEN AND HELL

Dear Lord

I have found you

Dear Lord

Hazar Imam

Opened the door

And let me in

Dear Lord

Hazar Imam

Reminded me

My day on earth

Confused with Angels Give A Tour Of Heaven
And Hell

Dear Lord

Hazar Imam

Said read

Angels Give A Tour Of Heaven And Hell To A
Soul

A=Angels Are Ordered By Allah

N=Now Let The Soul Decide

Moeze M Lalji

G=Ginans We Gave The Body

E=Enough We Have Spoken

L=Let The Tour Begin In Silence

S=Soul Will Know Who We Are

GIVE

G=Giving Up The Body Heaven Showed

I=Important Was The Forgiveness Ceremony

V=Very Few Souls Understood This

E=Every Resident Of Heaven Was Saying Forgive

A

A=All The Time You Cannot Sit By The Body

SCHIZOPHRENIA AND MULTICULTURALISM

TOUR

T=Trying To Settle Scores Of The Past

O=Only The Soul Was Too Hurt

U=Under Earth It Took Painful Experience

R=Remembered The Angels In Their Book

OF

O=Only God Understood The Soul

F=For God Ordered The Angel To Tour Hell

HEAVEN

H=Hell Was Shown To The Soul

E=Every Pain Received By The Soul

A=All Responsible Were Their

V=Visit Each One Said The Angel

E=Every Pain Of Yours Is Being Accounted By Your Lord

N=Not Until You Forgive They Remain Accounting Here

AND

A=And So The Soul Says God You Are You Are What You Are

N=Never Did I Know You Valued My Honest Pain

D=Did Every Tear Of My Body Matter To You

HELL 🥀

H=Heaven I Shall Enter Now Peacefully

E=Every Score Has Been Settled

L=Light Of Forgiveness Is From Heaven

L=Light Of Forgiveness Hell Cries Out For Every Painful Tear Caused On Earth

Dear Lord 🥀

You said learn from

Hazar Imam

The Heaven shall open

Amen 🥀

SCHIZOPHRENIA AND MULTICULTURALISM

IT IS NATURAL FOR YOUR HUSBAND

Dear Lord

I have found you

Dear Lord

Hazar Imam

Opened the door

And let me in

Dear Lord

Hazar Imam

Reminded me

My day on earth

Confused with It Is Natural For Your Husband

Dear Lord

Hazar Imam

Said read

IT IS NATURAL FOR YOUR HUSBAND

I=I Only Speak For The Husband

T=That What We Feel Is Natural For The Wife

IS

I=Important It Is To Make Love

S=Soul Is Making Love Through The Body

NATURAL

N=No We Can't Express This Love

A=Anywhere Else

T=Talim Of Allah Refuses

U=Under Marriage You Express Your Love

R=Remember Many Circumstances

A=Are There To Bring The Flame Of Love

L=Love Flame May Be Ignited By The Way You Said Something

SCHIZOPHRENIA AND MULTICULTURALISM

FOR 🌹

F=For The Love Flame Sometimes Has No Reason

O=Only Do Not Frustrate It

R=Respect It Wife If You Understand

YOUR 🌹

Y=You He Loves When He Sees A Beautiful Flower

O=Only He Wants To Hold You

U=Understand His Feelings

R=Respect It Wife If You Understand

HUSBAND 🌹

H=Have You Not Heard Positive Feelings

U=Understand Positive Feelings

S=Shame You Should Not Feel

B=But The Husband Becomes Quiet

A=And Withdrawn

N=No He Does Not Want To Make Love Under Force

D=Divine Is This Feeling Please Understand

Dear Lord

You said learn from

Hazar Imam

The Heaven shall open

Amen

DAUGHTER IN LAW 2

Dear Lord

I have found you

Dear Lord

Hazar Imam

Opened the door

And let me in

Dear Lord

Hazar Imam

Reminded me

My day on earth

Confused with Daughter in Law

Dear Lord

Hazar Imam

Said read

DAUGHTER IN LAW

D=Do respect her position

A=Away she has come from her family

U=Understand a new baby is born away from Allah

G=Give her the love of a new baby to bond

H=Heaven is born out of love

T=To reduce her anger love her

E=Everyday your son will be happy

R=Respect her like your daughter

IN

I=Important it is that you ring her

N=Never mind if she forgets to ring you

LAW

L=Little quarrels in a marriage means it is a good marriage

A=And parents should tell their son about this

W=When the son complains tell him it is nothing new

Dear Lord

SCHIZOPHRENIA AND MULTICULTURALISM

You said learn from

Hazar Imam

The Heaven shall open

Amen

WHAT SCIENCE CAN DO FOR YOU

Dear Lord

I have found you

Dear Lord

Hazar Imam

Opened the door

And let me in

Dear Lord

Hazar Imam

Reminded me

My day on earth

Confused with What Science Can Do For You

Dear Lord

Hazar Imam

Said read

WHAT SCIENCE CAN DO FOR YOU

W=Witness For You

H=How Things Work

SCHIZOPHRENIA AND MULTICULTURALISM

A=And Play With It

T=Throwing New Solutions

SCIENCE

S=Soul It Cannot Touch

C=Creator It Cannot Defeat

I=Iman It Cannot Understand

E=Eternal Life It Cannot Prove

N=Noor Of Allah It Keeps Out

C=Caught Out By The Quran

E=Eternal Life Is A Problem

CAN

C=Cancer It Can Cure
A=Allah It Is Still Understanding
N=Noor Of Allah It Is Still Understanding

FOR

F=Firmans Of Allah Made Science
O=Only Science Is Acting These Firmans
R=Room Of Science Is Good Deeds

YOU

Y=You Must Not Be Profit Motivated
O=Only You Were Created To Serve Mankind
U=Under Allah That Is Your Job Description
Dear Lord
You said learn from
Hazar Imam
The Heaven shall open
Amen

QUALITY EDUCATION

Dear Lord

I have found you

Dear Lord

Hazar Imam

Opened the door

And let me in

Dear Lord

Hazar Imam

Reminded me

My day on earth

Confused with Quality Education

Dear Lord

Hazar Imam

Said read

QUALITY EDUCATION

Q=Question The Right To Basic Needs

U=Understand Basic Needs For All

Moeze M Lalji

A=Are These Provided By Democracy

I=Important Is Housing

T=To Bring Up Stable Families

Y=You Cannot Abuse Human Rights Of Basic Needs

SCHIZOPHRENIA AND MULTICULTURALISM

EDUCATION

E=Every Government Is Looking For Taxes

D=Democracy Is For The People

U=Understand Basic Needs Are For The People

C=Can The Government Not Understand

A=All They Care For Is Taxes

T=The World Has To Unite

I=Impose A Human Rights Law On Abuse Of Basic Needs

O=Only Then Is Democracy For The People It Cares For

N=Now Is The Time To Help Our Children

Dear Lord

You said learn from

Hazar Imam

The Heaven shall open

Amen

WHAT BRITAIN CAN DO FOR ITS CHILDREN

Dear Lord 🌹

I have found you

Dear Lord 🌹

Hazar Imam

Opened the door

And let me in

Dear Lord 🌹

Hazar Imam

Reminded me

My day on earth

Confused with What Britain Can Do For Its
Children

Dear Lord 🌹

Hazar Imam

Said read

WHAT BRITAIN CAN DO FOR ITS CHILDREN 🌹

W=Wealth Of Britain Is Its Future Children

H=However Much You Spend

SCHIZOPHRENIA AND MULTICULTURALISM

A=All Is Not Enough

T=The Government Knows

BRITAIN

B=But Besides Education

R=Respect Needs To Be Given To Reality

I=Important It Is For Children

T=To See The Plight Of Poor Children and Families

A=All This In The Third World Countries

I=Important Is Real Exposure

N=Never Shelter Children In Classrooms

CAN

C=Can We Not Create An Education Budget

A=Allowing Children To Spend Time

N=Next To Reality Of Being Poor

DO

D=Do This For The Future Wealth Of Britain

O=Only Britain's Children Will Be Assertive

FOR

F=For Being Assertive Requires Experience

O=Only Classroom Experience

R=Removes Them From Real Understanding

ITS

I=Improve Their Field Training

T=To Make Them Responsible

S=So They Appreciate The Field

CHILDREN

C=Come In Time

H=Hear Children Appreciating Britain

I=Improving Creative Solutions To Problems

SCHIZOPHRENIA AND MULTICULTURALISM

L=Life Creative Solutions To World Life Problems

D=Deep Will Become Their Attitude

R=Respect They Will Have For People

E=Everyone Contributes With Real Sense

N=Never Should Children Be Sheltered

Dear Lord

You said learn from

Hazar Imam

The Heaven shall open

Amen

TONY BLAIR

Dear Lord

I have found you

Dear Lord

Hazar Imam

Opened the door

And let me in

Dear Lord

Hazar Imam

Reminded me

My day on earth

Confused with Tony Blair

Dear Lord

Hazar Imam

Said read Tony Blair

TONY BLAIR

T=Talk To Bush

O=Only To Rush Into Decisions

N=Never Has This Country Ignored Its
Government and People

SCHIZOPHRENIA AND MULTICULTURALISM

Y=You and Bush Have Created An Ocean Full Of Tears

BLAIR

B=Brother Hood Of Man In United Nations

L=Left It To One Side

A=Always Britain Has a Tradition Of Evolution

I=Ignoring History We Are All In Tears

R=Respect For Britain We Want Back In Evolution

Dear Lord

You said learn from

Hazar Imam

The Heaven shall open

Amen

I VISITED MY PARENTS TODAY

Dear Lord

I have found you

Dear Lord

Hazar Imam

Opened the door

And let me in

Dear Lord

Hazar Imam

Reminded me

My day on earth

Confused with I Visited My Parents Today

Dear Lord

Hazar Imam

Said read

I VISITED MY PARENTS TODAY

I=Important true story I listened

VISITED

V=Very important true story

I=In our relatives

SCHIZOPHRENIA AND MULTICULTURALISM

S=So I hope

I=Iman can grow

T=That Allah is in charge

E=Every minute he has planned

D=Dua we give to Allah and Noor of Allah

MY

M=Mother, family and community were upset

Y=Your daughter is deaf and dumb

PARENTS

P=Please break her relationship

A=As the boy is also deaf and dumb

R=Re-think for their children

E=Even they will be deaf and dumb

N=Never will Allah forgive us

T=The matter went before the doctors

S=So the doctors said let Allah decide why judge

SCHIZOPHRENIA AND MULTICULTURALISM

TODAY

T=Today they are married with two normal children

O=Only the children have learnt sign language

D=Devoted they are to their parents

A=Always have faith in Allah says my mother

Y=Your circumstances are in the hands of Allah says my mother

Dear Lord

You said learn from

Hazar Imam

The Heaven shall open

Amen

REPUBLIC OF IRAQ

Dear Lord
I have found you
Dear Lord
Hazar Imam
Opened the door
And let me in
Dear Lord
Hazar Imam
Reminded me
My day on earth
Confused with Republic of Iraq
Dear Lord
Hazar Imam
Said read
REPUBLIC OF IRAQ
R=Real Tears Feel Up An Ocean
E=Everyone Is In This Ocean
P=Patience Says The Quran

SCHIZOPHRENIA AND MULTICULTURALISM

U=Under The Quran This Is The Heart

B=Bridges Have To Be Built

L=Long Lasting Bridges Over The Ocean

I=In Tears We All Make One Ocean

C=Catch This Picture From The Soul Not The Mind

OF

O=Ocean Of Unity We Need

F=Forgive For Patience The Heart Of Quran

IRAQ

I=Iman You Must Not Loose IRAQ

R=Roshen Allah Do Not Loose IRAQ

A=Allah Do Not Loose IRAQ

Q=Quran Is The Heart Do Not Loose IRAQ

Dear Lord

You said learn from

Hazar Imam

The Heaven shall open

Amen

SCHIZOPHRENIA AND MULTICULTURALISM

IN HONOUR OF MY MOTHER AND FATHER

Dear Lord

I have found you

Dear Lord

Hazar Imam

Opened the door

And let me in

Dear Lord

Hazar Imam

Reminded me

My day on earth

Confused with In Honour of My Mother and
Father

Dear Lord

Hazar Imam

Said read

IN HONOUR OF MY MOTHER AND FATHER

I=Important you are in the hands of Allah

N=Noor of Allah holds you in his hands

HONOUR

H=Honour comes from the batuni world

O=Only the angels hold Allah's firmans

N=Never angels allow for parents to defend against their children

O=Only the angels hold Allah's firmans

U=Understand angels will correct you

R=Respect Allah commands through angels for what he holds in honour

OF

O=Only understanding is at fault

F=Firmans of Allah they forget

SCHIZOPHRENIA AND MULTICULTURALISM

MY

M=Many have travelled on this path

Y=You will not defeat what Allah holds in his hands in honour

MOTHER

M=Many said you were not educated

O=Others said you had a depressed background

T=They say you are the culprit of the house

H=How can we sit next to her many said

E=Explain to her what is status and how to sit in society they said

R=Respect Mother my mind lost for you by repeating the same words

AND

A=Allah my heart used to cry

N=No understanding did I have

D=Depression has brought me to see what Allah holds in his hands in honour

FATHER

F=Father all the words above were true for you

A=All was confusing in my mind

T=Times have been hard for you both

H=How my heart used to cry

E=Excellent you are in my heart always angels protect this firman by Allah

R=Respect Allah wants me to give to you by showing these words to His world

Dear Lord

You said learn from

Hazar Imam

The Heaven shall open

Amen

SCHIZOPHRENIA AND MULTICULTURALISM

GEORGE BUSH

Dear Lord

I have found you

Dear Lord

Hazar Imam

Opened the door

And let me in

Dear Lord

Hazar Imam

Reminded me

My day on earth

Confused with George Bush

Dear Lord

Hazar Imam

Said read

GEORGE BUSH

G=Giving is your country

E=Enterprising is your country

O=Only freedom you protect

R=Run too fast sometimes

G=Giving backfires

E=Enterprising backfires

BUSH

B=Backing away is a problem

U=Unity is what you are trying

S=Soul is definitely upset to see lots of deaths

H=How are we going to solve it

Dear Lord

You said learn from

Hazar Imam

The Heaven shall open

Amen

SCHIZOPHRENIA AND MULTICULTURALISM

DISCUSSION WITH MY WIFE

Dear Lord

I have found you

Dear Lord

Hazar Imam

Opened the door

And let me in

Dear Lord

Hazar Imam

Reminded me

My day on earth

Confused with Discussion With My Wife

Dear Lord

Hazar Imam

Said read

DISCUSSION WITH MY WIFE

D=Discuss blood is thicker than water

I=Important are parents

S=Soul cannot let go however hard you try

C=Catches your soul the bond all the time

U=Under bad parents this is the same

S=Soul of yours sees your parents as gold

S=Soul of mine sees my parents as gold

I=Important to you are your brothers they are gold

O=Only the soul cannot let go of the bond

N=No circumstances in between will change this feeling

SCHIZOPHRENIA AND MULTICULTURALISM

WITH

W=With your family you may have a dispute

I=Iman for your family will not go

T=Telling off your family by me all the time

H=Hell will become your heart it is natural

MY

M=My only choice in the matter

Y=You will want me to keep a distance for peace

WIFE

W=What does Idi Amin's son think of his dad

I=Important he is in his eyes despite what the world has seen

F=For it is important to understand the natural law

E=Everybody has to judge their relationship and decide on distance for peace

Surah 17:23 And your Lord has decreed that you worship none but Him. And that you be dutiful to your parents. If one of them or both of them attain old age in your life, say not to

them a word of disrespect, nor shout at them
but address them in terms of honour.

Surah 17:24 And lower unto them the wing of
submission and humility through mercy, and
say: `My Lord! Bestow on them Your Mercy as
they did bring me up when I was young.'

Dear Lord

You said learn from

Hazar Imam

The Heaven shall open

Amen

SCHIZOPHRENIA AND MULTICULTURALISM

REPUBLIC OF UGANDA

Dear Lord

I have found you

Dear Lord

Hazar Imam

Opened the door

And let me in

Dear Lord

Hazar Imam

Reminded me

My day on earth

Confused with Republic of Uganda

Dear Lord

Hazar Imam

Said read

REPUBLIC OF UGANDA

R=Respect we have for our motto `For God and My Country'

E=Excellent is our anthem `Oh Uganda, Land of Beauty'

P=President we all stand by

U=Under Prime Minister we all stand by

B=Better has become the country

L=Long gone is the revolution

I=In comes evolution for investment

C=Come and see Uganda

OF

O=Only Idi Amin we learn from

F=For revolution destroys progress

SCHIZOPHRENIA AND MULTICULTURALISM

UGANDA

U=Under the president

G=Growth is endless

A=All land is virgin

N=No man is lazy

D=Devotion is to Uganda

A=All people are ready for `Oh Uganda, Land of Beauty'

Dear Lord

You said learn from

Hazar Imam

The Heaven shall open

Amen

REPUBLIC OF KEYNA

Dear Lord

I have found you

Dear Lord

Hazar Imam

Opened the door

And let me in

Dear Lord

Hazar Imam

Reminded me

My day on earth

Confused with Republic of Kenya

Dear Lord

Hazar Imam

Said read

REPUBLIC OF KENYA

R=Respect we have for Harambee – Let us pull together

SCHIZOPHRENIA AND MULTICULTURALISM

E=Eternally we know Ee Mungu Nguvu Yetu –
Oh God of All Creation

P=President we all stand by

U=United we stand by

B=Better we want to make Kenya

L=Let there be no better country than Kenya

I=Important it is that the world knows

C=Come let us respect Kenya

OF

O=Only evolution helps

F=For revolution destroys progress

KENYA

K=Keep Keyna clean and safe

E=Every help it will receive

N=No-one can match your wildlife

Y=Your land is very attractive

A=Assets you have for peace

Dear Lord

You said learn from

Hazar Imam

The Heaven shall open

Amen

SCHIZOPHRENIA AND MULTICULTURALISM

UNITED REPUBLIC OF TANZANIA

Dear Lord

I have found you

Dear Lord

Hazar Imam

Opened the door

And let me in

Dear Lord

Hazar Imam

Reminded me

My day on earth

Confused with United Republic of Tanzania

Dear Lord

Hazar Imam

Said read

UNITED REPUBLIC OF TANZANIA

U=Uhuru na Umoja – Freedom and Unity

N=Next to the President and Government

I=Important they are

T=The People stand by

E=Ever seeking Uhuru na Umoja

D=Destiny is in Uhuru na Umoja

SCHIZOPHRENIA AND MULTICULTURALISM

REPUBLIC

R=Rest assured

E=Everyone is doing their best

P=People are good hearted

U=Under different circumstances

B=Better will become circumstances

L=Livelihood will become better

I=Investment is pouring in

C=Come and join Uhuru na Umoja

OF

O=Only God we believe in

F=For Mungu ibiriki Afrika – God Bless Africa

TANZANIA

T=Together is the answer

A=Always unity is the answer

N=Never mind the differences

Z=Zindaghi is differences

A=Always unity is the answer

N=Never bring revolution

I=Important is evolution for Uhuru na Umoja

A=Always evolution brings Mungu ibiriki Afrika

Dear Lord

You said learn from

Hazar Imam

The Heaven shall open

Amen

SCHIZOPHRENIA AND MULTICULTURALISM

UNITED KINGDOM

Dear Lord

I have found you

Dear Lord

Hazar Imam

Opened the door

And let me in

Dear Lord

Hazar Imam

Reminded me

My day on earth

Confused with United Kingdom

Dear Lord

Hazar Imam

Said read

UNITED KINGDOM

U=Under Her Majesty The Queen

N=Nation stands firm

I=Important is the system of Government

T=Takes into account democratic principles

E=Excellent is the respect for all

D=Democratic laws protect all

KINGDOM

K=Keeping hold on long traditions

I=Important is evolution

N=Nobody is hurt by evolution

G=Gone are the days of revolution

D=Demand not revolution

O=Only respect for each other is evolution

M=Mother earth unfolds gradually and blossoms

Dear Lord

You said learn from

Hazar Imam

The Heaven shall open

Amen

SCHIZOPHRENIA AND MULTICULTURALISM

WHAT MADE ME HAPPY

Dear Lord

I have found you

Dear Lord

Hazar Imam

Opened the door

And let me in

Dear Lord

Hazar Imam

Reminded me

My day on earth

Confused with What Made Me Happy

Dear Lord

Hazar Imam

Said read

WHAT MADE ME HAPPY

W=When good feelings come

H=House them

A=Always put them in action

T=Teach your family

MADE

M=My feelings said buy flowers and chocolates

A=And two sets I bought

D=Delivered one set to my wife as from me and my daughter

E=Explained to my daughter the next set was for her from me and mum

ME

M=Mother's Day it was

E=Excellent opportunity it was

SCHIZOPHRENIA AND MULTICULTURALISM

HAPPY

H=Happily my daughter questioned why for me

A=Always a daughter is a little mother I explained

P=Proud she felt

P=Proud she felt asking why mum

Y=Your mum I said is looking after me in my illness

Dear Lord

You said learn from

Hazar Imam

The Heaven shall open

Amen

TODAY'S THERAPY SAYS I AM A GOOD HUSBAND

Dear Lord

I have found you

Dear Lord

Hazar Imam

Opened the door

And let me in

Dear Lord

Hazar Imam

Reminded me

My day on earth

Confused with Today's Therapy Says I Am A Good Husband

Dear Lord

Hazar Imam

Said read

TODAY'S THERAPY SAYS I AM A GOOD HUSBAND

T=Take my daughter to school everyday

O=Only to bring her back afterwards

SCHIZOPHRENIA AND MULTICULTURALISM

D=Daily I can cook if need be

A=Always taking the burden off my wife

Y=You have to understand what she has gone through

THERAPY

T=Together we are taught to cope

H=Have your feelings expressed to each other

E=Enforce them not

R=Respect each others feelings

A=Always learn to compromise

P=Previous feelings are an experience

Y=You can build on your experience

SAYS

S=Say you are a good husband

A=Always say you are a good wife

Y=You both shall remain together

S=Say nothing good Allah destroys

SCHIZOPHRENIA AND MULTICULTURALISM

I

I=I take you forever and forever

AM

A=Always we should wait for understanding

M=Mowla says evolution not revolution

A

A=Any relationship has problems

GOOD

G=Give and take we do because our love is eternal

O=Only Allah knows our good intentions

O=Only Mowla knows our good intentions

D=Dua will make us see our good intentions

HUSBAND

H=Held each other in good and bad times

U=Under bad times we have not divorced

S=So in good times we have not divorced

B=By no means a mistress I have

A=All your wishes I hold even if I have to cry

N=Never I command knowledge over you

D=Deep down nothing will come with us except faith given by Mowla

Dear Lord

You said learn from

Hazar Imam

The Heaven shall open

Amen

SCHIZOPHRENIA AND MULTICULTURALISM

ALCOHOL SMOKING DRUGS

Dear Lord

I have found you

Dear Lord

Hazar Imam

Opened the door

And let me in

Dear Lord

Hazar Imam

Reminded me

My day on earth

Confused with Alcohol Smoking Drugs

Dear Lord

Hazar Imam

Said read

ALCOHOL SMOKING DRUGS

A=Allah says do not drink

L=Light of Allah conveys the message

C=Catch the message if you can

O=Only if you want to sit next to Mowla

H=Have no excuses for Day of Judgement

O=Only your mind you want to listen to

L=Light of Allah you must get closer to

SMOKING

S=Soul is crying give up

M=Mowla is crying give up

O=Only Allah is unhappy

K=Kick the habit

I=Iman has to grow

N=Now spend that money on your mother

G=Grave will open paradise for you

DRUGS

D=Dua and dasond I keep you away from

R=Roshni of Allah I have taken

U=Under the Light of Allah I have removed you from

G=Ginans I have taken from you

S=Soul has no value except mind I teach

Dear Lord

You said learn from

SCHIZOPHRENIA AND MULTICULTURALISM

Hazar Imam

The Heaven shall open

Amen

SOME OF MY SYMPTOMS OF DEPRESSION

Dear Lord

I have found you

Dear Lord

Hazar Imam

Opened the door

And let me in

Dear Lord

Hazar Imam

Reminded me

My day on earth

Confused with Some Of My Symptoms Of Depression

Dear Lord

Hazar Imam

Said read

SOME OF MY SYMPTOMS OF DEPRESSION

S=Shouting and being abusive at my wife on any little thing

SCHIZOPHRENIA AND MULTICULTURALISM

O=Only feeling that my brain can take no more information

M=Many paranoid thoughts go through the brain and voices I hear

E=Even thinking my parents and family have plotted against me

OF

O=Only became emotional with whatever my wife said

F=Find myself writing emotional poetry and crying

MY

M=Many times I hit the wall and doors

Y=Yes I even broke the car windscreen because my wife said something

SYMPTOMS

S=So it was all triggered by the closure of our Post Office on fraud charge

Y=Yet it took seven years to go to court to prove we were honest

M=Money compensation was £15,000 which we sent back

P=Personal history of depression exists in my family with suicide

T=Talking about the way you feel in depression is the hardest

O=Only at this stage you do not want to be alive and faith is gone

M=Mowla made me attend therapy groups and doors opened slowly

S=Soon you see others in similar or different situations talking to therapists

OF

O=Only talk if you want to there is no pressure whatsoever

F=For the main thing is you have come out of the house

DEPRESSION

SCHIZOPHRENIA AND MULTICULTURALISM

D=Do tell your therapist even if you have transport problems

E=Everybody's depression is different based on circumstances

P=Personally I had to accept that I have a chemical imbalance in the brain

R=Respect your therapist will give you no matter what you feel or think

E=Even I found expressing by fax to my psychiatrist was helpful

S=Sending emails to my social worker was helpful

S=Speaking to a 24hour help line by mental health team was helpful

I=Important are these steps to ease pressure on my wife or your family

O=Only talk to mental health team about depression they can cope and support you

N=Never mind if you do not feel socialising but let your family enjoy their lives

Dear Lord

You said learn from

Hazar Imam

The Heaven shall open

Amen

DURING THE PERIODS OF MY DEPRESSION

Dear Lord

I have found you

Dear Lord

Hazar Imam

Opened the door

And let me in

Dear Lord

Hazar Imam

Reminded me

My day on earth

Confused with `During the periods of my depression'

Dear Lord

Hazar Imam

Said read

SCHIZOPHRENIA AND MULTICULTURALISM

DURING THE PERIODS OF MY
DEPRESSION

D=Death is all the mind could show me

U=Understanding was lost

R=Removed from iman by the mind

I=Important was death to the mind

N=Nor could I understand myself

G=Given up to the voices of death

THE

T=Took myself to the doctor

H=How was I to explain

E=Everything I wrote for the doctor and cried

PERIODS

P=Psychiatrist I went to see

E=Explained my feelings by crying

R=Removed from work by the psychiatrist

I=Immediately medication I started

O=Only at home I would sleep

D=Despair I was not wanting anybody

S=Soul would cry in small flames to Mowla and
Allah

OF

O=Only supported by my wife and mental health team

F=For my daughter was too small – 5 years of age

MY

M=Mowla and Allah you have to understand now

Y=You understand Mowla and Allah now

SCHIZOPHRENIA AND MULTICULTURALISM

DEPRESSION

D=Death my mind was crying to Mowla and Allah

E=Everytime a picture would come in my mind

P=Picture had Mowla sitting on his chair

R=Removed I would be from death by this picture

E=Everytime Mowla would make me sit next to him by his feet

S=See how much close you are to me Mowla would say

S=See nobody is allowed here except you Mowla would say

I=Important is your iman Allah brings you here he would say

O=Only sit next to me with your highest qualification iman he would say

N=Nothing else you need to look at I am here Mowla would say

Dear Lord

You said learn from

Hazar Imam

The Heaven shall open

Amen

SCHIZOPHRENIA AND MULTICULTURALISM

WHY BLAME THE MOTHER ONLY

Dear Lord

I have found you

Dear Lord

Hazar Imam

Opened the door

And let me in

Dear Lord

Hazar Imam

Reminded me

My day on earth

Confused with Why Blame The Mother Only

Dear Lord

Hazar Imam

Said read

WHY BLAME THE MOTHER ONLY

W=When the house falls blame the mother only

H=House is in a problem blame the mother only

Y=You please understand mother only

BLAME

B=Begin with the most beautiful mother only

L=Life is full of love with the most beautiful mother only

A=Arrive children with the most beautiful mother only

M=Mother is ignored only

E=Everyone loves the children from the most beautiful mother only

SCHIZOPHRENIA AND MULTICULTURALISM

THE

T=Then the story changes with the most beautiful mother only

H=House grows with stress with the most beautiful mother only

E=Every stress is on the most beautiful mother only

MOTHER

M=Mother has no support from the husband

O=Over the children there is no control

T=They choose bad company

H=House is in chaos

E=Everyone blames the most beautiful mother only

R=Respect is lost by the most beautiful mother only

ONLY

O=Only think for the most beautiful mother

N=Never leave her alone in the battlefield

L=Learn both of you how to manage a family

Y=You both are the most beautiful make the family the most beautiful by support

Dear Lord

You said learn from

Hazar Imam

The Heaven shall open

Amen

SCHIZOPHRENIA AND MULTICULTURALISM

MARY HAD A LITTLE LAMB

Dear Lord

I have found you

Dear Lord

Hazar Imam

Opened the door

And let me in

Dear Lord

Hazar Imam

Reminded me

My day on earth

Confused with Mary Had A Little Lamb

Dear Lord

Hazar Imam

Said read

MARY HAD A LITTLE LAMB

M=Mary I must say is our lovely wife

A=Always you will be her lamb

R=Respect this Mother Nature feeling

Y=You are her lamb don't laugh

HAD

H=Have respect for this rope

A=All married man have this rope

D=Damage it you will stray

A

A=Always pull gentle on the rope

SCHIZOPHRENIA AND MULTICULTURALISM

LITTLE

L=Like your mother she holds you

I=It is siratalmustaquim (the straight road)

T=Talk to Mary if you want to go out

T=Tell Mary of all your moves

L=Let there be trust in the rope

LAMB

L=Little Lamb you are not to loose

A=Always the lamb she loves

M=Many times there will be push and pull on the rope

B=Be gentle on the rope it is siratalmustaquim

Dear Lord

You said learn from

Hazar Imam

The Heaven shall open

Amen

Moeze M Lalji

DAUGHTER IN LAW

Dear Lord
I have found you
Dear Lord
Hazar Imam
Opened the door
And let me in
Dear Lord
Hazar Imam
Reminded me
My day on earth
Confused with Daughter In Law
Dear Lord
Hazar Imam
Said read

DAUGHTER IN LAW

D=Demand not the same
A=Always blood is thicker than water

SCHIZOPHRENIA AND MULTICULTURALISM

U=Understand your position

G=Give not hatred

H=Have your feelings understood

T=Take a back step if it is complicated

E=Even let your husband know

R=Remember your husband cannot cut off from his parents

IN

I=If it is physical and mental cruelty

N=Never accept it

LAW

L=Let your husband see his parents

A=And you go to your parents

W=With time let understanding prevail for peace

Dear Lord

You said learn from

Hazar Imam

The Heaven shall open

Amen

SCHIZOPHRENIA AND MULTICULTURALISM

POLLY PUT THE KETTLE ON

Dear Lord 🐿
I have found you
Dear Lord 🐿
Hazar Imam
Opened the door
And let me in
Dear Lord 🐿
Hazar Imam
Reminded me
My day on earth
Confused with Polly Put The Kettle On
Dear Lord 🐿
Hazar Imam
Said read

POLLY PUT THE KETTLE ON 🐿
P=Please remember to put the kettle on
O=Only remember your wife needs a break

L=Lighten her burden

L=Learn if a break helps use it

Y=You know your circumstances well

PUT

P=Please send your wife to her family

U=Understand her needs

T=Take it from me I have learnt

SCHIZOPHRENIA AND MULTICULTURALISM

THE

T=The cement between the two should not harden

H=Hard cement allows no breathing space

E=Every relationship needs oxygen

KETTLE

K=Keep to this and see the benefits

E=Every child you will look after

T=Telephone you will daily to your wife

T=Telephone you will daily to say you miss her

L=Life you will see from her point of view

E=Even your children will learn to cook

ON

O=Only Polly Put The Kettle On For Your Wife

N=Never goes wasted an experience

Dear Lord

You said learn from

Hazar Imam

The Heaven shall open

Amen

SCHIZOPHRENIA AND MULTICULTURALISM

VISIT YOUR MOTHER

Dear Lord

I have found you

Dear Lord

Hazar Imam

Opened the door

And let me in

Dear Lord

Hazar Imam

Reminded me

My day on earth

Confused with visit your mother

Dear Lord

Hazar Imam

Said read

VISIT

V=Visit Your Mother

I=Improve The Relationship

S=Send Her Flowers

I=Improve The Relationship

T=Try And Understand

YOUR

Y=You Are Her Branch Of Tree

O=Only You Listen

U=Understand This

R=Respect Means You Are Her Branch Of Tree

SCHIZOPHRENIA AND MULTICULTURALISM

MOTHER

M=Mother Your Mother

O=Only If You Understand

T=Tell Her Not She Is Bad

H=Heaven She Will Still Keep Open

E=Ever Green She Is

R=Respect Her You Will Have Respected
Father And Noor of Allah

Dear Lord

You said learn from

Hazar Imam

The Heaven shall open

Amen

MY BROTHER

Dear Lord

I have found you

Dear Lord

Hazar Imam

Opened the door

And let me in

Dear Lord

Hazar Imam

Reminded me

My day on earth

Confused with My Brother

Dear Lord

Hazar Imam

Said read

MY

M=May we remain forever under GOD's blessings

Y=You and I come under GOD's blessings

SCHIZOPHRENIA AND MULTICULTURALISM

BROTHER

B=Before marriage we were with mum and dad under GOD's blessings

R=Remember the car toys given by mum and dad under GOD's blessings

O=Only you protected me as told by mum and dad under GOD's blessings

T=Tears made me innocent in front of mum and dad under GOD's blessings

H=How circumstances change in front of mum and dad under GOD's blessings

E=Emotions change with circumstances in front of mum and dad under GOD's blessings

R=Remember but the car toys given by mum and dad under GOD's blessings

Dear Lord

You said learn from

Hazar Imam

The Heaven shall open

Amen

TWINKLE TWINKLE LITTLE STARS

Dear Lord

I have found you

Dear Lord

Hazar Imam

Opened the door

And let me in

Dear Lord

Hazar Imam

Reminded me

My day on earth

Confused with Twinkle Twinkle Little Stars

Dear Lord

Hazar Imam

Said read

TWINKLE TWINKLE LITTLE STARS

T=Twinkle Twinkle Little Stars

W=What are Twinkle Twinkle Little Stars

I=Important they are Twinkle Twinkle Little Stars

SCHIZOPHRENIA AND MULTICULTURALISM

N=Noor of Allah keeps blessing Twinkle Twinkle Little Stars

K=Kind you have to be to Twinkle Twinkle Little Stars

L=Love your Twinkle Twinkle Little Stars

E=Educate your Twinkle Twinkle Little Stars

TWINKLE

T=Twinkle Twinkle Little Stars

W=When little introduce them numbers

I=In early age introduce them reading

N=Never will they be scared of numbers

K=Kind they will be to reading

L=Let them not loose on the internet

E=Early habits matter the most Twinkle Twinkle Little Stars

LITTLE

L=Learn them not to be frightened of asking questions in class

I=Important habit it is in class and home

T=Tell them to question is to learn

T=Tell them to question is to understand

L=Let them know problems build up

E=Ending in a mountain to be sorted out requiring tears

STARS

S=So those who ask become Twinkle Twinkle Little Stars

T=Take care of this simple habit to become Twinkle Twinkle Little Stars

A=Assertiveness they learn to become Twinkle Twinkle Little Stars

R=Review the habit daily to become Twinkle Twinkle Little Stars

S=Soon they will drive on this habit to be Twinkle Twinkle Little Stars Up Above The World So High With the Grace of Mowla and Allah

SCHIZOPHRENIA AND MULTICULTURALISM

Dear Lord

You said learn from

Hazar Imam

The Heaven shall open

Amen

PLEASE DO NOT DO THIS EVER I CRY

Dear Lord

I have found you

Dear Lord

Hazar Imam

Opened the door

And let me in

Dear Lord

Hazar Imam

Reminded me

My day on earth

Confused with Please Do Not Do This Ever I Cry

Dear Lord

Hazar Imam

Said read

PLEASE DO NOT DO THIS EVER I CRY

P=Please do not do this ever I cry

L=Life before marriage – I cry

SCHIZOPHRENIA AND MULTICULTURALISM

E=Endlessly I worked for my boyfriend from overseas – I cry

A=All financial support I gave to my love to become a lawyer – I cry

S=Soon he qualified we married – I cry

E=Entered in our lives two beautiful sons – I cry

DO

**D=Devoted was my husband to his business –
I cry**

O=Only to fall in love with his secretary – I cry

NOT

**N=Next on their honeymoon they phone me – I
cry**

O=Only to say `I divorce you' – I cry

T=They had a Muslim marriage – I cry

DO

D=Devasted I became – I cry

**O=Only my wife was there to support her – I
cry**

THIS

**T=Tears and emotional breakdown my wife
held – I cry**

H=House became divorced – I cry

**I=Immediately she left for another country – I
cry**

SCHIZOPHRENIA AND MULTICULTURALISM

S=Support she took from her parents and sisters – I cry

EVER

E=Endlessly she works to support her two children – I cry

V=Visited her but numb she is – I cry

E=Even the husband is now crying with his second family – I cry

R=Remember do not do this to any woman Allah places in your hands – I cry

I

I=Inspite of this she allows the children to visit their father – I cry

CRY

C=Comfort she receives attached to Mowla with her tasbi – I cry

R=Remember she has forgiven her husband and wants him not – I cry

Y=You who read this freewill is in your hands – I cry

Dear Lord

You said learn from

Hazar Imam

The Heaven shall open

Amen

SCHIZOPHRENIA AND MULTICULTURALISM

TALK WITH MY NEIGHBOUR

Dear Lord

I have found you

Dear Lord

Hazar Imam

Opened the door

And let me in

Dear Lord

Hazar Imam

Reminded me

My day on earth

Confused with Talk with my neighbour

Dear Lord

Hazar Imam

Said read

TALK WITH MY NEIGHBOUR

T=Talking with my good English neighbour

A=Always religion seems to be a problem he said

L=Life has become divided over religion he said

K=Keeping family united over religion does not work he said

WITH

W=When will we have respect for each other he said

I=Important were parents but this is changing he said

T=Tell your children anything they leave house he said

H=Hold them for respect they rebel he said

MY

M=My days you took your hat off to respect elders he said

Y=Youth today you fear to say anything he said

SCHIZOPHRENIA AND MULTICULTURALISM

NEIGHBOUR

N=Not only are you facing this I said

E=Every culture is going in this direction slowly I said

I=Importance to human values of brotherhood are going I said

G=Give a thought to Adam and Eve I said

H=Has anybody got the time to remember them I said

B=Best parents of all mankind which cannot be denied I said

O=Only if mankind would give honour in each house I said

U=Under honour I mean a photograph of Adam and Eve in every house I said

R=Respect for Adam and Eve makes us brothers we both agreed

Dear Lord

You said learn from

Hazar Imam

The Heaven shall open

Amen

DAY OF JUDGEMENT

Dear Lord

I have found you

Dear Lord

Hazar Imam

Opened the door

And let me in

Dear Lord

Hazar Imam

Reminded me

My day on earth

Confused with Day of Judgement

Dear Lord

Hazar Imam

Said read

DAY OF JUDGEMENT

D=Day only my Lord knows the Day

A=All those with freewill will stand up on the
Day

SCHIZOPHRENIA AND MULTICULTURALISM

Y=You have no choice in the matter on the Day

OF

O=Only Angels will lay open your book on the Day

F=Freedom you will not have to hire lawyers on the Day

JUDGEMENT

J=Judges will see how to judge on the Day

U=Understand Angels will present your case on the Day

D=Doubts will not be raised on what Angels present on the Day

G=Ginans of Hazar Imam in your record will be praised on the Day

E=Erasing your record will not be allowed on the Day

M=Mowla will not be allowed to come in between on the Day

E=Eternal life you denied and your mischief is present on the Day

N=Noor of Allah you denied and your mischief is present on the Day

T=Take care of this world, repent and make no mischief to see on the Day

Dear Lord 🥀

You said learn from

Hazar Imam

The Heaven shall open

Amen

SCHIZOPHRENIA AND MULTICULTURALISM

LET US LOOK AT THE STARS

Dear Lord

I have found you

Dear Lord

Hazar Imam

Opened the door

And let me in

Dear Lord

Hazar Imam

Reminded me

My day on earth

Confused with Let Us Look At The Stars

Dear Lord

Hazar Imam

Said read

LET US LOOK AT THE STARS

L=Look they have been placed so high up by Allah

E=Everyone must look as lovers do but not touch

T=Time has gone by nobody can bring them down

U=Understand the deeper meaning

S=Search for a promise to bring them down nobody can

L=Look on earth everybody is a star

O=Only on earth everybody has free will

O=Only the stars do not have freewill

K=Keep this in mind

A=Allah knows the weakness in man

T=Tell him about free will he runs away from his position

H=He runs destroying other stars

E=Everytime there is chaos on Earth

S=Stars how peaceful you are without freewill

T=Talim us mankind for peace

SCHIZOPHRENIA AND MULTICULTURALISM

A=Allah or take away the freewill so the Earth is heavenly like the stars

R=Respecting freewill is too much for mankind

S=Stars you were clever, you knew freewill was temporary as the material world, an illusion for chaos and a heavy responsibility taken by man from God

Dear Lord

You said learn from

Hazar Imam

The Heaven shall open

Amen

MY FATHER

Dear Lord

I have found you

Dear Lord

Hazar Imam

Opened the door

And let me in

Dear Lord

Hazar Imam

Reminded me

My day on earth

Confused with MY Father

Dear Lord

Hazar Imam

Said read

MY

M=My father I did not understand until I experienced FATHERHOOD

Y=You will not understand fatherhood until you experience FATHERHOOD

SCHIZOPHRENIA AND MULTICULTURALISM

FATHER

F=Father Allah has made you like the SUN

A=Allah knows the SUN burns HOT so he made it to SHINE

T=Take care the SUN further shines through the cool blue SKY to EARTH

H=Hold your FAMILY by shining on your wife whose status is that of EARTH

E=Eternally your wife has your children's paradise at her FEET

R=Roshni of Allah is with your wife as she is EARTH

Dear Lord

You said learn from

Hazar Imam

The Heaven shall open

Amen

MY HUSBAND

Dear Lord

I have found you

Dear Lord

Hazar Imam

Opened the door

And let me in

Dear Lord

Hazar Imam

Reminded me

My day on earth

Confused with My Husband

Dear Lord

Hazar Imam

Said read

MY

M=May we remain forever under Allah's blessings

Y=You and I have met under Allah's blessings

SCHIZOPHRENIA AND MULTICULTURALISM

HUSBAND

H=Hug each other daily under Allah's blessings

U=Under Allah barkat is received for my wife under Allah's blessings

S=Say that we will comfort each others feelings under Allah's blessings

B=Build no barriers with each other under Allah's blessings

A=Away we will keep bad habits under Allah's blessings

N=Never we will hurt each other over our parents under Allah's blessings

D=Dua and tasbi we will say together daily under Allah's blessings

WITH ALL MY LOVE, YOUR DEAREST HUSBAND xxxxx

Dear Lord

You said learn from

Hazar Imam

The Heaven shall open

Amen

MY WIFE

Dear Lord
I have found you
Dear Lord
Hazar Imam
Opened the door
And let me in
Dear Lord
Hazar Imam
Reminded me
My day on earth
Confused with My Wife
Dear Lord
Hazar Imam
Said read

MY

M=May we remain forever under Allah's
blessings

SCHIZOPHRENIA AND MULTICULTURALISM

Y=You and I have met under Allah's blessings

WIFE

W=Witnesses are Angels under Allah's blessings

I=Important it is we hold each other under Allah's blessings

F=For if my wife is happy the house is happy under Allah's blessings

E=Even if Allah gives us no children we can adopt under Allah's blessings

WITH All MY LOVE, YOUR DEAREST WIFE xxxx

Dear Lord

You said learn from

Hazar Imam

The Heaven shall open

Amen

MARRIAGE

Dear Lord

I have found you

Dear Lord

Hazar Imam

Opened the door

And let me in

Dear Lord

Hazar Imam

Reminded me

My day on earth

Confused with Marriage

Dear Lord

Hazar Imam

Said read

MARRIAGE

M=Many excuses Allah creates to bring BOTH OF YOU TOGETHER

A=Angels just carry out the farmans to bring BOTH OF YOU TOGETHER

SCHIZOPHRENIA AND MULTICULTURALISM

R=Respect Allah and his farmans to bring
BOTH OF YOU TOGETHER

R=Remember your circumstances are perfect
to bring BOTH OF YOU TOGETHER

I=Invest now in honesty and trust to keep
BOTH OF YOU TOGETHER

A=Allah shows you marriage you both have to
run it to keep BOTH OF YOU

TOGETHER

G=Giving and taking are accepted without
counting to keep BOTH OF YOU

TOGETHER

E=Every wife talks more than the husband to
keep BOTH OF YOU TOGETHER

Dear Lord

You said learn from

Hazar Imam

The Heaven shall open

Amen

SENSITIVE PERSON

Dear Lord

I have found you

Dear Lord

Hazar Imam

Opened the door

And let me in

Dear Lord

Hazar Imam

Reminded me

My day on earth

Confused with Sensitive Person

Dear Lord

Hazar Imam

Said read

SENSITIVE

S=Soul thinks about everybody but itself

E=Everybody has to be pleased

N='No' is difficult to say afraid it might hurt feelings

SCHIZOPHRENIA AND MULTICULTURALISM

S=Soul builds stress in the mind

I=Iman in Jamat gets difficult with coping with people

T=Talim becomes too engrossed looking for answers

I=Iman in Hazar Imam becomes one of crying

V=Visiting your parents and family becomes difficult

E=Eternal soul needs help and support to learn to say `No'

PERSON

P=Please talk about your feelings with your support

E=Everyone in life is imperfect

R=Respect yourself first by talking your feelings with your support

S=Slowly and slowly you will learn to say `No'

O=Only then you will be in charge of yourself

N=Never will you enjoy life under `Yes', Allah and Hazar Imam also says `NO'

Dear Lord

You said learn from

Hazar Imam

The Heaven shall open

Amen

SCHIZOPHRENIA AND MULTICULTURALISM

FLOWERS

Dear Lord

I have found you

Dear Lord

Hazar Imam

Opened the door

And let me in

Dear Lord

Hazar Imam

Reminded me

My day on earth

Confused with Flowers

Dear Lord

Hazar Imam

Said read

FLOWERS

F=Freedom to Blossom they Say

L=Love they want to Shine

O=Only love they want to Give

W=Witness the colours and perfumes they want to Express

E=Eternally they want to be like This

R=Remember they want to be Happy

S=So Hazar Imam says I am happy with my Jamat I bless them to be Flowers

Dear Lord

You said learn from

Hazar Imam

The Heaven shall open

Amen

SCHIZOPHRENIA AND MULTICULTURALISM

HUG YOUR MOTHER

Dear Lord

I have found you

Dear Lord

Hazar Imam

Opened the door

And let me in

Dear Lord

Hazar Imam

Reminded me

My day on earth

Confused with Hug Your Mother

Dear Lord

Hazar Imam

Said read

HUG YOUR MOTHER 🌹

HUG 🌹

H=Happy she will BE

U=Understand her NOT

G=Giving is all she DOES

G=Giving is all she DOES

YOUR 🌹

Y=You are her BABY

O=Only you she PROTECTS

U=Understand her NOT

R=Remembers you ONLY

SCHIZOPHRENIA AND MULTICULTURALISM

MOTHER

M=Mother she IS

O=Only you she PROTECTS

T=Teach her NOT

H=Has paradise under her FEET

E=Eternity she will show YOU

R=Respect is well overdue to HER

Dear Lord

You said learn from

Hazar Imam

The Heaven shall open

Amen

MOTHER

Dear Lord

I have found you

Dear Lord

Hazar Imam

Opened the door

And let me in

Dear Lord

Hazar Imam

Reminded me

My day on earth

Confused with Mother

Dear Lord

Hazar Imam

Said read

SCHIZOPHRENIA AND MULTICULTURALISM

MOTHER

M=Mother and Earth hold the highest status in front of MOWLA and ALLAH

O=Only Mother will HOLD YOU what may come in her LAP

T=Tell people off if she finds on YOU even a drop of RAIN

H=Hold you even if YOU become independent in her LAP

E=Eternally by HER feet lies paradise placed by ALLAH and she knows through BIRTH

R=Roshni of Allah she will make sure YOU receive even by placing TEARS at night to Mowla and Allah which YOU never see until your WIFE becomes a MOTHER

Dear Lord

You said learn from

Hazar Imam

The Heaven shall open

Amen

CHILDREN

Dear Lord

I have found you

Dear Lord

Hazar Imam

Opened the door

And let me in

Dear Lord

Hazar Imam

Reminded me

My day on earth

Confused with Children

Dear Lord

Hazar Imam

Said read

SCHIZOPHRENIA AND MULTICULTURALISM

CHILDREN

C=CUDDLE the soul like the Angels did before bringing them to you

H=HUG the soul like the Angels did before bringing them to you

I=IGNORE the soul CRIES you will hear for Angels love

L=LOVE the soul like the Angels did before bringing them to you

D=DEGRADE the soul HURT you will hear for Angels protection

R=REMEMBER the soul forever like the Angels do

E=EDUCATE the soul like the Angels did before bringing them to you

N=NOOR OF ALLAH was the Light the soul was held under by the Angels

N=NOOR OF ALLAH was the LIGHT OF CUDDLE before BIRTH

N=NOOR OF ALLAH was the LIGHT OF HUG before BIRTH

N=NOOR OF ALLAH was the LIGHT OF LOVE before BIRTH

N=NOOR OF ALLAH was the LIGHT THAT REMEMBERS before BIRTH

N=NOOR OF ALLAH was the LIGHT OF EDUCATION before BIRTH

N=NOOR OF ALLAH children MISS

N=NOOR OF ALLAH is from ALLAH

N=NOOR OF ALLAH is how ALLAH HOLDS US

N=NOOR OF ALLAH is with the soul NOT BORN

N=NOOR OF ALLAH is with the soul BORN

N=NOOR OF ALLAH is with the soul DEPARTED

N=NOOR OF ALLAH is in THREE DIMENSIONS HOLDING ALL SOULS with ANGELS

Dear Lord

You said learn from

Hazar Imam

The Heaven shall open

Amen

SCHIZOPHRENIA AND MULTICULTURALISM

OCEAN

Dear Lord

I have found you

Dear Lord

Hazar Imam

Opened the door

And let me in

Dear Lord

Hazar Imam

Reminded me

My day on earth

Confused with Ocean

Dear Lord

Hazar Imam

Said read

OCEAN

O=Only by Allah's Farmans Angels take a DROP

C=Catch a drop with Allah's BLESSINGS

E=Eternal it becomes with Allah's BLESSINGS

A=Allah's blessings gives it birth and death to EXPERIENCE

N=Noor of Allah holds the drop for COMFORT for it feels LOST

Dear Lord

You said learn from

Hazar Imam

The Heaven shall open

Amen

SCHIZOPHRENIA AND MULTICULTURALISM

EARTH

Dear Lord

I have found you

Dear Lord

Hazar Imam

Opened the door

And let me in

Dear Lord

Hazar Imam

Reminded me

My day on earth

Confused with Earth

Dear Lord

Hazar Imam

Said read

EARTH

E=Everyone she carries without CRYING

A=Allah's Farmans she obeys to hold her TEARS

R=Remembers every pain that you give HER

H=Happy she will be on Day of Judgement releasing her TEARS

Dear Lord

You said learn from

Hazar Imam

The Heaven shall open

Amen

SCHIZOPHRENIA AND MULTICULTURALISM

RELIGION

Dear Lord

I have found you

Dear Lord

Hazar Imam

Opened the door

And let me in

Dear Lord

Hazar Imam

Reminded me

My day on earth

Confused with Religion

Dear Lord

Hazar Imam

Said read

RELIGION

R=Roshni of Creator to respect SHINES

E=Eternal Soul SHINES

L=Light of Creator SHINES

I=Iman to Respect creation SHINES

G=Ginans to Love each other SHINES

I=Iman to Forgive each other SHINES

O=Only the Creator we have to account
SHINES

N=Noor of Creator is Peace for mankind
SHINES

Dear Lord

You said learn from

Hazar Imam

The Heaven shall open

Amen

SCHIZOPHRENIA AND MULTICULTURALISM

ISLAM AND PLURALISM

Dear Lord

I have found you

Dear Lord

Hazar Imam

Opened the door

And let me in

Dear Lord

Hazar Imam

Reminded me

My day on earth

Confused with Islam

Dear Lord

Hazar Imam

Said read

I=Iman: Brotherhood of man truthfully say
'There is or there isn't a God'

S=Soul: Brotherhood of man truthfully says
'Let me find out or not'

L=Light of Understanding (Noor): Brotherhood
of man truthfully read, listen, talk, see, feel and
write

A=Allah is happy because Brotherhood of Man truthfully give a Pluralistic view

M=Mowla is happy because Brotherhood of Man truthfully agree with his understanding to live United Under Pluralism

Dear Lord

You said learn from

Hazar Imam

The Heaven shall open

Amen

SCHIZOPHRENIA AND MULTICULTURALISM

YOU CAN BUY THIS IN THE MARKET!!!!!

Dear Lord

I have found you

Dear Lord

Hazar Imam

Opened the door

And let me in

Dear Lord

Hazar Imam

Reminded me

My day on earth

Confused with A Funny Story

Dear Lord

Hazar Imam

Said read

A FUNNY STORY

A= A Little Daughter Saw Her Father

FUNNY

F=Father She Saw In The Bathroom

U=Under The Shower

N=Now She Was Puzzled

N=Now She Went Straight To Mummy

Y=You Know Mum What I Saw She Said

STORY

S=Something Hanging On Dad

T=Tell Me Mum Why I Do Not Have The Same

O=Only I Want The Same As Dad

R=Replied Mum Don't Worry Honey I Will Buy You One

Y=You Come With Me To The Market Tomorrow!!!!

Dear Lord

You said learn from

SCHIZOPHRENIA AND MULTICULTURALISM

Hazar Imam

The Heaven shall open

Amen

Moeze M Lalji

Golden jubilee 30 Go Children For Education

Dear Lord

I have found you

Dear Lord

Hazar Imam

Opened the door

And let me in

Dear Lord

Hazar Imam

Reminded me

My day on earth

Confused with Golden Jubilee

Dear Lord

Hazar Imam

Said read

SCHIZOPHRENIA AND MULTICULTURALISM

GOLDEN JUBILEE

G=Go For Education Children

O=Only Be Motivated

L=Life Always Has Problems

D=Do Not Let Them Build Up

E=Everyday At School

N=Never Sit On A Problem

JUBILEE

J=Just A Mountain Of Problems Will Rise

U=Understand You Will Cry and Give Up

B=Better Start On Good Habits

I=Immediately Seek Help for Solutions

L=Little Excuse You Have Nowadays

E=Eventually Your Good Habit Will Bring Success

E=Eventually Your Good Habit Will Bring Success

Dear Lord

You said learn from

Hazar Imam

The Heaven shall open

Amen

SCHIZOPHRENIA AND MULTICULTURALISM

GOLDEN JUBILEE POEM O MOWLA

Dear Lord

I have found you

Dear Lord

Hazar Imam

Opened the door

And let me in

Dear Lord

Hazar Imam

Reminded me

My day on earth

Confused with O Mowla

Dear Lord

Hazar Imam

Said read

O Mowla 🌹
When You Will Come
On Your Golden Jubilee

O Mowla 🌹
When You Will Come
On Your Golden Jubilee
I Will Be Bowed Down

O Mowla 🌹
On Your Golden Jubilee
I Will Be Bowed Down
Light Of Allah I Will Be Seeing

O Mowla 🌹
On Your Golden Jubilee
Light Of Allah I Will Be Seeing
Light That Has Travelled Since Adam

SCHIZOPHRENIA AND MULTICULTURALISM

O Mowla

On Your Golden Jubilee

Light That Has Travelled Since Adam

My Body Will Disappear

O Mowla

On Your Golden Jubilee

My Body Will Disappear

My Body Will Take All Its Tears

O Mowla

On Your Golden Jubilee

My Body Will Take All Its Tears

Because The Light Of Allah Loves All

O Mowla

On Your Golden Jubilee

Because The Light Of Allah Loves All

No More Will The False Voices Torment Me

O Mowla

On Your Golden Jubilee

No More Will The False Voices Torment Me

No More Will The False Eyes Look Down On Me

O Mowla

On Your Golden Jubilee

No More Will The False Eyes Look Down On Me

SCHIZOPHRENIA AND MULTICULTURALISM

No More Will My Mental Status Be Unloved

O Mowla

On Your Golden Jubilee

No More Will The False Eyes Look Down On Me

No More Will My Mental Status Be Unloved

O Mowla

On Your Golden Jubilee

No More Will My Mental Status Be Unloved

No More Will My Family Turn Away From Me

O Mowla 🌹

On Your Golden Jubilee

No More Will My Family Turn Away From Me

No More Will My Wife Have To Cry In The World

O Mowla 🌹

On Your Golden Jubilee

No More Will My Wife Have To Cry In The World

No More Will The Jamat See Falsehood

O Mowla 🌹

On Your Golden Jubilee

No More Will The Jamat See Falsehood

Only The Soul And Light Of Allah Will Be One In Allah's Love

O Mowla 🌹

On Your Golden Jubilee

SCHIZOPHRENIA AND MULTICULTURALISM

Only The Soul And Light Of Allah Will Be One In Allah's Love

Only The Soul And Light Of Allah Will Be One In Allah's Love

Dear Lord

You said learn from

Hazar Imam

The Heaven shall open

Amen

Golden jubilee 25 Go To A Baby

Dear Lord

I have found you

Dear Lord

Hazar Imam

Opened the door

And let me in

Dear Lord

Hazar Imam

Reminded me

My day on earth

Confused with Golden Jubilee

Dear Lord

Hazar Imam

Said read

SCHIZOPHRENIA AND MULTICULTURALISM

GOLDEN JUBILEE

G=Go To A Baby

O=Only To Be Born In A Garden Of Human-beings

L=Left Alone Without A Flower To See

D=Development Will Be Without Reflection

E=Every Ethics Comes From Reflection

N=Now The Baby Sees A Beautiful Flower

JUBILEE

J=Joy The Baby Will Bring To The Garden Of Human-beings

U=Understand Joy The Baby Will Bring To The Garden

B=Because The Fragrance Of Pure God

I=Is Good Deeds For The Human Garden

L=Let The Baby See The Flower In The Human Garden

E=Every Regret You Will Have If You Remove The Flower

E=Every Regret You Will Have If You Remove The Flower

175

Dear Lord

You said learn from

Hazar Imam

The Heaven shall open

Amen

SCHIZOPHRENIA AND MULTICULTURALISM

WHAT IS A WOMAN

Dear Lord

I have found you

Dear Lord

Hazar Imam

Opened the door

And let me in

Dear Lord

Hazar Imam

Reminded me

My day on earth

Confused with What Is A Woman

Dear Lord

Hazar Imam

Said read

WHAT IS A WOMAN

W=WORDS GO WITH WOMEN

H=HAS TO EXPRESS MORE WORDS THAN A MAN

A=ALLAH WANTS MORE WORDS FROM A WOMAN

T=THIS IS ALL CONFIRMED BY SCIENCE AND WHAT WE SEE

IS

I=IMPORTANT IS HER BRAIN FOR MULTI-TASK

S=SHE CAN HANDLE MORE INSTRUCTIONS AT THE SAME TIME

SCHIZOPHRENIA AND MULTICULTURALISM

A

A=A MAN'S BRAIN CANNOT COPE WITH TOO MANY INSTRUCTIONS

WOMAN

W=WOMAN GIVE YOUR MAN ONE INSTRUCTION AT A TIME

O=ONLY TOO MUCH BLOWS HIS BRAIN

M=MAKE A LIST FOR HIS BRAIN TO COPE

A=A WOMAN NEEDS TO GET HER WORDS OUT OTHERWISE SHE FEELS LOW

N=NOW MAN UNDERSTAND SHE IS NOT SHOOTING YOU!!!! SHE STILL LOVES YOU!!!!YOU BOTH NEED TO UNDERSTAND WHAT ALLAH HAS CREATED

Dear Lord

You said learn from

Hazar Imam

The Heaven shall open

Amen

Dear Lord

I have found you

Dear Lord

Hazar Imam

Opened the door

And let me in

Dear Lord

Hazar Imam

Reminded me

My day on earth

Confused with If You Cannot Handle Your Wife

Dear Lord

Hazar Imam

Said read

SCHIZOPHRENIA AND MULTICULTURALISM

IF YOU CANNOT HANDLE YOUR WIFE

I=If You Cannot Handle Your Wife

F=For Divorce Is Not The Answer

YOU

Y=You Understand One Wife

O=Only Then You Will Understand Every Wife

U=Understand One Wife

CANNOT

C=Catch Allah In Your Understanding

A=Allah Is Calling You To Understand His Creation

N=No Point Running Away

N=No Point Running Away

O=Only Bowing Down To Understanding

T=Talim Is What You Need

HANDLE

H=Houses All Over The World

A=All Have Problems

N=No Experience Is Without Pain

D=Deepen Your Understanding

L=Love Allah's Creation And You Have Found Allah

E=Every Faithfull Husband Has Tears

YOUR

Y=You Do Not Own Your Wife

O=Only Allah Is Her Master

U=Understand Her Root Problem Is Insecurity

R=Respect It With Love Saying Allah Is There

WIFE

W=When She Cries Hold Her Tears Don't React

I=If She Is Angry Be Like My Brother Don't React Smile

F=For Any Pain She Brings Out Understand By Holding It

SCHIZOPHRENIA AND MULTICULTURALISM

E=Every Wife Is The Same They Need To
Express Not A Divorce

Dear Lord

You said learn from

Hazar Imam

The Heaven shall open

Amen

Golden jubilee 9

Pluralism

Dear Lord

I have found you

Dear Lord

Hazar Imam

Opened the door

And let me in

Dear Lord

Hazar Imam

Reminded me

My day on earth

Confused with Golden Jubilee

Dear Lord

Hazar Imam

Said read

GOLDEN JUBILEE

G=Good Deeds Are Increasing

O=Only The World Knows

L=Light Of Allah Keeps Shining Good Deeds

D=Deeds For Humanity

E=Every Human Being Will Be Under Good Deeds

N=No More Will The World Be Selfish

JUBILEE

J=Just The Nature Of The Heart

U=Understands Good Deeds

B=But The Beauty Is Pluralism

I=Important Is Pluralism

L=Light Of Good Deeds Is In Pluralism

E=Every Good Deed Comes From Pluralism

E=Every Good Deed Comes From The Garden Of Pluralism

Dear Lord

You said learn from

Hazar Imam

The Heaven shall open

Amen

SCHIZOPHRENIA AND MULTICULTURALISM

I took my dear on a white horse

Dear Lord

I have found you

Dear Lord

Hazar Imam

Opened the door

And let me in

Dear Lord

Hazar Imam

Reminded me

My day on earth

Confused with I Took My Dear On A White Horse

Dear Lord

Hazar Imam

Said read

I TOOK MY DEAR ON A WHITE HORSE 🌹

I=I Took My Dear On A White Horse From Heaven

TOOK 🌹

T=Took My Dear On A White Horse From Heaven

O=Only She Was Holding Onto Me From Heaven

O=Only She Was Holding Onto Me From Heaven

K=King Of Believers Blessed Us From Heaven

MY 🌹

M=Master I Was Of The White Horse From Heaven

Y=You Were Holding Onto Me From Heaven

DEAR 🌹

D=Death Could Not Touch The White Horse From Heaven

E=Every Gate Was Open For The White Horse From Heaven

SCHIZOPHRENIA AND MULTICULTURALISM

A=Allah's Firman Open The White Gates Of Heaven

R=Receive Angels The White Horse From Heaven

ON

O=Only Protect The White Horse From Heaven

N=No Couple Should Come Off The White Horse From Heaven

A

A=Allah's Firman On The White Horse From Heaven

WHITE

W=White Horse From Heaven reaches Earth

H=Holding Of The White Horse Has Changed

I=Important Rights Women Have Claimed

T=The White Horse They Ride As Well

E=Every White Horse Can Have A Husband Holding On

HORSE

H=Have Turns Riding The White Horse From Heaven

O=Only To Suit The Circumstances Of Earth

R=Respect Is There For The White Horse From Heaven

S=So Don't Be Surprised

E=Every White Horse Rides Differently According To Circumstances

Dear Lord

You said learn from

Hazar Imam

The Heaven shall open

Amen

SCHIZOPHRENIA AND MULTICULTURALISM

We met in the garden of prayer

 Dear Lord

I have found you

Dear Lord

Hazar Imam

Opened the door

And let me in

Dear Lord

Hazar Imam

Reminded me

My day on earth

Confused with We Met In The Garden Of Prayer

Dear Lord

Hazar Imam

Said read

WE MET IN THE GARDEN OF PRAYER

W=We Have Met In Different Circumstances

E=Every Circumstance Is Different

MET

M=Make It Your Garden Of Roses

E=Every Circumstance Is A Garden Of Roses

T=Take In The Beautiful Colours Of Love

IN

I=Important Is To Remember The Colours Of Love

N=Nearly Every Colour Of Love Was Breath Taking

THE

T=There Was The Fresh Colour Of The Face

H=Hugging Was A Strong Colour Of Love

E=Embracing Was A Strong Colour Of Love

SCHIZOPHRENIA AND MULTICULTURALISM

GARDEN

G=Giving Attention To Every Word Was A New Colour Of Love

A=Always Missing The Colours Of Love

R=Roshni Was In The Colours Of Love

D=Divine Was Each Colour Of Love

E=Eternal Was Each Colour Of Love

N=Noor Was Each Colour Of Love

OF

O=Only Your Garden Was Yours Full Of Roses

F=Freedom Of Love Was In The Bed Of Roses

PRAYER

P=Prayer Is May The Garden Of Love

R=Respect You Into Eternity

A=Always May The Garden Have Hugs

Y=Your Hugs Carry You Into Roses Of Eternity

E=Every Hug Is A Symbol Of Respect To Allah

R=Respect Every Hug Will Receive By Allah

Dear Lord

You said learn from

Hazar Imam

The Heaven shall open

Amen

SCHIZOPHRENIA AND MULTICULTURALISM

Money cannot buy you love

 Dear Lord

I have found you

Dear Lord

Hazar Imam

Opened the door

And let me in

Dear Lord

Hazar Imam

Reminded me

My day on earth

Confused with Money Cannot Buy Love

Dear Lord

Hazar Imam

Said read

MONEY CANNOT BUY LOVE

M=Mowla Does Not Want Your Money

O=Only Allah Made Money For His Love

N=Noor Of Allah Does Not Want Your Money

E=Eternal Soul Uses Money For Allah's Love

Y=Your Money Is Allah's Money For Allah's Love

CANNOT

C=Catch Allah With Your Money

A=Allah's Love You Can Take With You

N=Noor Of Allah You Can Take With You

N=Noor Of Allah You Can Take With You

O=Only Allah Gives Money To Know Him

T=The Grave And Money Belong To Allah To Love Him

SCHIZOPHRENIA AND MULTICULTURALISM

BUY 🥀

B=Better Understand

U=Under Mind Your Soul Receives Love Of Duniya Only

Y=You Mind Under Soul Receives Love Of Din And Duniya

LOVE 🥀

L=Love Your Soul To Love Your Mind

O=Only Then Money Will Give You Love For Din And Duniya

V=Visit Money To Buy You Love For Allah

E=Eternal Love Is Our Destiny With Allah

Dear Lord 🥀

You said learn from

Hazar Imam

The Heaven shall open

Amen 🥀

DEAR MEMBERS I DO NOT WANT TO OFFEND YOU

I WRITE POETRY AS A RESULT OF MY ILLNESS

I SUFFER FROM SCHIZOPHERNIA

THE POETRY LAYOUT IS FROM MY ISMAILI FAITH

IT CAME TO ME WHILE I WAS CRYING TO ALLAH AND HAZAR IMAM

AND IT IS VERY PART OF MY SOUL

POETRY REPRESENTS WHO I AM

AND IT SHOULD NO LONGER BE A CRIME

TO SAY THIS IS WHAT YOU ARE

I AM A HUMAN BEING SHARING MY EXPERINCE OF THE WORLD

FROM MY CORNER OF MY CIRCUMSTANCES GIVEN BY ALLAH

I DO NOT WANT MEMBERS TO BE OFFENDED BY MY POETRY

THAT IS NOT THE INTENTION

IF YOU ALL ARE OFFENDED THAN FOR PEACE

ALLAH WILL SAY STOP

AND CONSIDER ANOTHER STYLE

SCHIZOPHRENIA AND MULTICULTURALISM

IN PEACE I BOW DOWN TO ALL MEMBERS
YA ALI MADAT
MOEZE LALJI

IMAGINE YOUR BIRTH

Dear Lord

I have found you

Dear Lord

Hazar Imam

Opened the door

And let me in

Dear Lord

Hazar Imam

Reminded me

My day on earth

Confused with Imagine Your Birth

Dear Lord

Hazar Imam

Said read

IMAGINE YOUR BIRTH

I=Imagine you are born you are unaware - this is birth

M=Meaningless it is as you are unaware - this is birth

SCHIZOPHRENIA AND MULTICULTURALISM

A=All is provided as you are unaware - this is birth

G=Grow a little play all day unaware - this is birth

I=Ignore the world all day unaware – this is birth

N=Next your senses grow you become aware – this is birth

E=Enter your teenage years you become aware – this is birth

YOUR

Y=Your body is learning to take charge you become aware – this is birth

O=Only you have to talk now without mum you become aware – this is birth

U=Understand you have to drive now you become aware – this is birth

R=Respecting you have to drive now you become aware – this is birth

BIRTH

B=Best were the times you learnt from your parents unaware – this is birth

I=Improve your driving by reading road signals you are aware – this is birth

R=Respect other drivers on the road you are aware – this is birth

T=Take lessons about the road as it is endless you are aware – this is birth

H=Hold lessons with Hazar Imam so you don't keep driving unaware – this is birth

Dear Lord

You said learn from

Hazar Imam

The Heaven shall open

Amen

114 AREAS WHERE HAZAR IMAM AND GOD CAN GET UPSET

Dear Lord

I have found you

Dear Lord

Hazar Imam

Opened the door

And let me in

Dear Lord

Hazar Imam

Reminded me

My day on earth

Confused with 114 Areas Where Hazar Imam And Allah Can Get Upset

Dear Lord

Hazar Imam

Said read

114 AREAS WHERE HAZAR IMAM AND ALLAH CAN GET UPSET 🐑

1. **Not Respecting My Mother**

2. **Not Respecting My Mother**

3. **Not Respecting My Mother**

4. **Not Respecting My Mother**

5. **Not Respecting My Father**

6. **Not Respecting My Wife**

7. **Not Respecting My Wife's Family**

8. **Not Respecting My Husband**

9. **Not Respecting My Husband's Family**

10. **Not Respecting My Adopted Children**

11. **Not Respecting My Children**

12. **Not Respecting My Neighbours**

13. **Not Respecting My Daughter-In-Law**

14. **Not Respecting My Son-In-Law**

15. **Not Respecting My Granddaughters**

16. **Not Respecting My Grandsons**

17. **Not Respecting My Sisters**

18. **Not Respecting My Brothers**

19. **Not Respecting My Relatives**

20. **Not Respecting My Work Colleagues**

SCHIZOPHRENIA AND MULTICULTURALISM

21. Not Respecting Jamat Khanna

22. Not Respecting Hazar Imam's Institutions

23. Not Respecting All Religions

24. Not Respecting All Human Beings

25. Not Respecting My Health

26. Not Respecting My Health By Taking Alcohol

27. Not Respecting My Health By Taking Drugs

28. Not Respecting My Health By Taking Cigarettes

29. Not Respecting My Health By Not Taking Medication

30. Not Respecting My Mental Health By Not Taking Therapy

31.Not Respecting My Mental Health By Not Taking Medication

32. Not Respecting My Mental Health By Not Taking Holiday Breaks

33. Not Respecting My Soul

34. Not Respecting Eternal Life

35. Not Respecting Evolution In Life

36. Not Respecting Dialogue

37. Not Respecting Understanding

38. Not Respecting Compromise

39. Not Respecting Good Deeds

40. Not Respecting To Encourage Others Into Good Deeds

41. Not Respecting Charity Begins At Home

42. Not Respecting The Poor

43. Not Respecting The Widow

44. Not Respecting Unfortunate Circumstances Of Others

45. Not Respecting Making This World A Better Place Than You Found It In

46. Not Respecting Life Long Learning

47. Not Respecting The Truth

48. Not Respecting Making A Honest Living

49. Not Respecting Sharing Excess Wealth Given By Allah

50. Not Respecting Good Manners

51. Not Respecting Talking Softly

52. Not Respecting Being Assertive

53. Not Respecting Talking Your Feelings

54. Not Respecting Taking Good Advice

55. Not Respecting Sharing Your Problems

56. Not Respecting Seeking Solutions To Problems

57. Not Respecting That Life Is A Struggle

58. Not Respecting That Daily We Face New Problems

59. Not Respecting That Daily We Need Courage

60. Not Respecting That Daily We Need To Talk

61. Not Respecting That Everyone Has Problems

62. Not Respecting Other Peoples Property

63. Not Respecting Other Peoples Feelings

64. Not Respecting The Environment

65. Not Respecting The Country You Live In

66. Not Respecting The Laws Of That Country

67. Not Respecting The Culture Of That Country

68. Not Respecting The Democratic Rights Given To You

69. Not Respecting The Good Habits Of That Country

70. Not Respecting Living And Non Living Things

71. Not Respecting Building Bridges With Communities

72. Not Respecting Being Creative

73. Not Respecting Being Creative To Seek New Solutions

74. Not Respecting Allah's Creation

75.Not Respecting That Mankind Is Vicegerent On Earth

76. Not Respecting That Allah Wants No Mischief

77. Not Respecting Not To Suppress The Poor

78. Not Respecting Not To Suppress The Weak

79. Not Respecting Marriage Of Choice

80.Not Respecting Daughter's Choice Of Marriage

81. Not Respecting Son's Choice Of Marriage

82. Not Respecting The Time You Are In

83, Not Respecting The Circumstances You Are In

84. Not Respecting That Tomorrow Never Comes

85. Not Respecting That Things Have To Be Done Today

86. Not Respecting That Tomorrow You May Die

87. Not Respecting That Daughters Need Education

88. Not Respecting That Daughters May Need To Work

89. Not Respecting That Daughters Cannot Be Locked

90. Not Respecting That Time Changes

91. Not Respecting Balance Between Din And Duniya

92. Not Respecting To Roshen Allah

93. Not Respecting The Orphan

94. Not Respecting The Orphan's Property

95. Not Respecting The Orphan's Rights

96. Not Respecting Any Funeral And The Departed Souls

97. Not Respecting Voluntary Service – Work No Words

98. Not Respecting Giving Lifts To Momins With No Transport

99. Not Respecting Solving Problems For Momins

100. Not Respecting Offering Help Before Asked To Do So

101. Not Respecting Mukhishaeb

102. Not Respecting Kamadiashaeb

103. Not Respecting Mukhianima

104. Not Respecting Kamadianima

105. Not Respecting Volunteers

106, Not Respecting Council Members

107.Not Respecting Jamat Momins

108. Not Respecting Quran

109. Not Respecting Firmans

110. Not Respecting Ginans

111. Not Respecting Panj Tan Pak

112. Not Respecting Prophet Muhammad

113. Not Respecting Hazar Imam

114. Allah Has Given Above Instructions Through Mowla And Through Mowla I Can Ask Forgiveness To Amend To Become A Better Person It Does Not Make Mowla Allah. Allah Counts Your Intentions To Respect His Creation To Respect Him. Any Religion Or Human Being That Respects His Creation Respects The Creator. This Is What Angels Record From Me My Niyat (INTENTION)

Dear Lord

You said learn from

SCHIZOPHRENIA AND MULTICULTURALISM

Hazar Imam

The Heaven shall open

Amen

QUALITY EDUCATION 2

Dear Lord

I have found you

Dear Lord

Hazar Imam

Opened the door

And let me in

Dear Lord

Hazar Imam

Reminded me

My day on earth

Confused with Quality Education

Dear Lord

Hazar Imam

Said read

QUALITY EDUCATION

Q=Question The Right To Basic Needs

U=Understand Basic Needs For All

A=Are These Provided By Democracy

I=Important Is Housing

T=To Bring Up Stable Families

Y=You Cannot Abuse Human Rights Of Basic
Needs

EDUCATION

E=Every Government Is Looking For Taxes

D=Democracy Is For The People

U=Understand Basic Needs Are For The People

C=Can The Government Not Understand

A=All They Care For Is Taxes

T=The World Has To Unite

I=Impose A Human Rights Law On Abuse Of Basic Needs

O=Only Then Is Democracy For The People It Cares For

N=Now Is The Time To Help Our Children

Dear Lord

You said learn from

Hazar Imam

The Heaven shall open

Amen

SCHIZOPHRENIA AND MULTICULTURALISM

WHAT MY WIFE DOES NOT UNDERSTAND

Dear Lord

I have found you

Dear Lord

Hazar Imam

Opened the door

And let me in

Dear Lord

Hazar Imam

Reminded me

My day on earth

Confused with What My Wife Does Not
Understand

Dear Lord

Hazar Imam

Said read

WHAT MY WIFE DOES NOT UNDERSTAND

W=Wife Was Born In Karachi 1952

H=Had My Birth In Uganda 1958

A=And Our Adopted Daughter Born In Karachi 1992

T=These Factors Unite In England

MY

M=My Understanding Is Allah Plans For All

Y=You Can See It From The Above

WIFE

W=Wife Claims She Knew She Was Coming To England

I=Important Progress She Was Going To Make

F=For She Says One Must Have Will Power

E=Everything Depends On Your Motivation She Says

SCHIZOPHRENIA AND MULTICULTURALISM

DOES

D=Did She Know She Was Going To Adopt After Miscarriages

O=Only Allah Knew I Say

E=Even The House We Have Now

S=Say Only Allah Knew I Say

NOT

N=Never Know The Story Of The Book

O=Only Allah Knows Its Every Word

T=Think Over It My Dear Wife

UNDERSTAND

U=Understand The Loss Of Post Office Business

N=No Time Was Being Given To Our Daughter

D=Danger Was Growing Up Without Mum's Love

E=Every Daughter Must Grow Up With Mum

R=Respect The Lord's Decision

S=See He Care's For Daughters

T=Time Now Is Spent By Mum Looking After Daughter

A=Allah Has Rewarded You More Than The Business

N=Never Ignore Allah In Any Equation

D=Dua We Should Give To Allah And Hazar Imam For Our Daughter

Dear Lord

You said learn from

Hazar Imam

The Heaven shall open

Amen

SCHIZOPHRENIA AND MULTICULTURALISM

JAMAT KHANNA

Dear Lord

I have found you

Dear Lord

Hazar Imam

Opened the door

And let me in

Dear Lord

Hazar Imam

Reminded me

My day on earth

Confused with Jamat Khanna

Dear Lord

Hazar Imam

Said read

JAMAT KHANNA

J=Jamat

A=Allah Jamat Believes In

M=Mowla Jamat Believes In

A=Allah's Present Mowla Is Hazar Imam

T=Talim Of Jamat Is Under Hazar Imam

SCHIZOPHRENIA AND MULTICULTURALISM

KHANNA

K=Keep's Hazar Imam In Charge

H=House Of The Prophet Panj Tan Pak, Quran, Ginans and Hazar Imam Jamat Accepts

A=All Spiritual Authority Is Vested In Hazar Imam

N=Noor Of Allah Was In The Prophethood

N=Noor Of Allah Is Now In Hazar Imam

A=Allah's Light Of Allah Is Hazar Imam

Dear Lord

You said learn from

Hazar Imam

The Heaven shall open

Amen

HOW TO REPLY TO YOUR MOTHER

Dear Lord

I have found you

Dear Lord

Hazar Imam

Opened the door

And let me in

Dear Lord

Hazar Imam

Reminded me

My day on earth

Confused with How to reply to your mother

Dear Lord

Hazar Imam

Said read

HOW TO REPLY TO YOUR MOTHER

H=Hug her

O=Only she understands your hug

W=Witness she knows

SCHIZOPHRENIA AND MULTICULTURALISM

TO

T=Tell her you love her

O=Only she will hold you by the ear

REPLY

R=Respect this sweet action

E=Encourage her by saying it is spiritual barkat

P=Please tell me off for more spiritual barkat

L=Light of Allah will be pleased

Y=You will carry this eternally

YOUR 🌹

Y=You only have to smile

O=Only the smile we will take

U=Understand mother is sweet

R=Respect this sweet with a smile for heaven

MOTHER 🌹

M=Mother tell me off

O=Only I know it leads to spiritual barkat

T=The more you tell us off the more spiritual barkat we get

H=Hell closes with more spiritual barkat

E=Every door of heaven will be opened by Angels

R=Respect is all your family will receive from Angels

Dear Lord 🌹

You said learn from

Hazar Imam

The Heaven shall open

Amen 🌹

www.ingramcontent.com/pod-product-compliance
Lightning Source LLC
Chambersburg PA
CBHW031506270326
41930CB00006B/282